Colonoscopy
FOR

DUMMIES®

SPECIAL EDITION

by Kathleen Dobie

Carol Burke, MD, Technical Editor

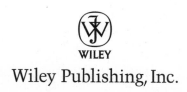

WILEY

Wiley Publishing, Inc.

Colonoscopy For Dummies® Special Edition

Published by
Wiley Publishing, Inc.
111 River Street
Hoboken, NJ 07030-5774
www.wiley.com

Copyright © 2011 by Wiley Publishing, Inc., Indianapolis, Indiana

Published by Wiley Publishing, Inc., Indianapolis, Indiana

For general information on our other products and services, please contact our Business Development Department in the U.S. at 317-572-3205. For details on how to create a custom For Dummies book for your business or organization, contact info@dummies.biz. For information about licensing the For Dummies brand for products or services, contact BrandedRights&Licenses@Wiley.com.

ISBN: 978-0-470-61661-1

Manufactured in the United States of America

10 9 8 7 6 5 4 3 2

WILEY

About the Author

Kathleen Dobie is an established freelance writer and editor. Her 30-year career in publishing includes selling and writing books as well as editing of all kinds — copyediting, development editing, and project editing. She is the go-to writer for *For Dummies* custom health titles; her credits include *HSAs For Dummies, Lasik Surgery For Dummies,* and *Navigating Your Health Benefits For Dummies.*

About the Technical Editor

Carol Burke, MD, is the Director of the Center for Colon Polyp and Cancer Prevention in the Department of Gastroenterology and Hepatology at the Cleveland Clinic. Through 20 years of gastroenterology practice, Dr. Burke has balanced her passion for treating patients with colorectal cancer prevention research.

Dr. Burke is internationally known for her work in the hereditary colorectal cancer syndromes and research on the use of agents to prevent colon polyps and cancer. Her research funding includes the National Cancer Institute, Department of Defense, Industry, and the American College of Gastroenterology, to name a few.

She is past chair of the American College of Gastroenterology Educational Affairs Committee, Women in Gastroenterology Committee, and is currently on the Board of Trustees. She is past assistant editor of the American Journal of Gastroenterology, has authored numerous peer reviewed manuscripts, abstracts, and book chapters, and is a frequent reviewer for many digestive disease journals.

Publisher's Acknowledgments

We're proud of this book and of the people who worked on it. For details on how to create a custom For Dummies book for your business or organization, contact info@dummies.biz. For details on licensing the For Dummies brand for products or services, contact BrandedRights&Licenses@Wiley.com.

Some of the people who helped bring this book to market include the following:

Acquisitions, Editorial, and Media Development

Project Editor: Jennifer Bingham

Editorial Manager: Rev Mengle

Business Development Representative: Melody Layne

Custom Publishing Project Specialist: Michael Sullivan

Composition Services

Project Coordinator: Kristie Rees

Layout and Graphics: SDJumper

Proofreader: Lindsay Littrell

Special Help: Hennie Hasson, Cleveland Clinic; Jeff Driggs, Salix Pharmaceuticals; Landy Townsend, Salix Pharmaceuticals; Bil Boyd, MedThink Communications; Greg O'Donnell, MedThink Communications

Publishing and Editorial for Technology Dummies

    Andy Cummings, Vice President and Publisher

Publishing and Editorial for Consumer Dummies

    Diane Graves Steele, Vice President and Publisher, Consumer Dummies

    Kristin Ferguson-Wagstaffe, Product Development Director, Consumer Dummies

    Ensley Eikenburg, Associate Publisher, Travel

    Kelly Regan, Editorial Director, Travel

Composition Services

    Debbie Stailey, Director of Composition Services

Business Development

    Lisa Coleman, Director, New Market and Brand Development

Contents at a Glance

Table of Contents

Introduction

· ·

Colonoscopy has long suffered from a bad rap, but the reputation isn't deserved. Sure, you may feel fear, embarrassment, anger — a whole host of emotions when facing the recommendation by your physician to have a colonoscopy. But, the truth is that the vast majority of colonoscopy patients don't have a terrible experience. Some don't remember the procedure at all. (The bowel prep process is a different story, but just look at that as time out of your life spent in the worthy cause of trying to prolong it.)

The simple truth is that a colonoscopy may be one of the essential steps you take for your good health, like eating right and exercising.

Colonoscopy is usually recommended as a colon cancer screening test. Colonoscopy has been shown to prevent colorectal cancer, which is the second leading cause of cancer and cancer-related deaths in men and women in America. According to the Centers for Disease Control and Prevention, 60 percent of deaths from colorectal cancer could be prevented if everyone age 50 and older were screened regularly.

 If you don't want to have a colonoscopy for yourself, do it for your family. Nothing is more heartbreaking than to watch someone you love slip away from you. Especially when a colonoscopy would have prevented colon cancer.

About This Book

If you're reading this book, there's a good chance that you have been told you need a colonoscopy. Perhaps when confronted with the reality of facing colonoscopy, your reaction was less than excited. This is very natural.

I wrote this book to ease your anxiety about getting a colonoscopy. I address some common (and some not-so-common) questions you may have about the colonoscopy experience.

I tell you what a colonoscopy is, why your healthcare provider may have told you that you need to get one, and the best way to prepare for one. I discuss the most common fears and misconceptions associated with getting a colonoscopy.

I trust that you'll soon recognize that a colonoscopy isn't nearly as bad as you think. The fact is that a colonoscopy is a vital, potentially life-saving procedure.

If you have questions about the colonoscopy procedure or your health, there is no substitute for an honest discussion with your healthcare provider. Before receiving an order for your colonoscopy and a prescription for your colonoscopy preparation, discuss the following with your doctor: your medical history, your current condition, and the medications and dietary supplements that you are taking (prescription and over-the-counter).

How to Use This Book

In this book, I try to give you all the information you need on a specific topic in one place. I divide the book into chapters as follows and hope that the titles tell you what's in each:

- ✔ Chapter 1: Understanding What a Colonoscopy Is and Why to Get One
- ✔ Chapter 2: Looking at Colorectal Cancer
- ✔ Chapter 3: Planning for Your Colonoscopy
- ✔ Chapter 4: Explaining the Bowel Prep Process
- ✔ Chapter 5: Experiencing the Colonoscopy Procedure
- ✔ Chapter 6: Getting Back to Normal after Your Colonoscopy
- ✔ Chapter 7: Ten Common Questions
- ✔ Chapter 8: Ten (Okay, Seven) Uncommon Questions

I *italicize* defined terms and highlight some information with an icon in the margin.

Icons Used in This Book

Throughout this book, I use several helpful little icons in the margins.

Information to keep in mind as you go through the colonoscopy process is marked with this stringed finger.

If you have questions, consult your healthcare provider, especially about topics highlighted with this icon.

The bullseye marks information you can make use of.

Chapter 1

Understanding What a Colonoscopy Is and Why to Get One

*I*f you have been scheduled to have a colonoscopy, congratulations on taking an important step in caring for your health.

Explaining the What and Why of Colonoscopy

A colonoscopy is a quick (usually less than 30 minutes), wholly or mostly painless procedure that is usually performed on an outpatient basis. Procedures can be done at the hospital's outpatient department or in your physician's ambulatory surgery center, and you go back home the same day.

Examining the procedure

A *colonoscopy* is a common procedure in which a healthcare professional, usually a gastroenterologist, examines the entire inner lining of the large intestine, which includes the colon and rectum. The examination is done to check for *polyps* (pronounced *pawl*-ips), abnormal growths that can grow into cancer, as well as to diagnose other gastrointestinal problems such as inflammation and bleeding.

During the colonoscopy, the doctor inserts a thin, flexible, lighted tube, called a *colonoscope,* into the anus and through the colon until it reaches the *cecum,* the area where the small and large intestine meet. The colonoscope allows your doctor to inflate your colon with air, cleanse the surface lining with water, inspect the lining for abnormalities, take photographs and tissue samples, and remove polyps. (I explain the whole procedure in Chapter 5.)

Because of its shape, location in the body, and the fact that its internal walls are lined with many recesses and folds, the colon is tricky to examine. The best way to do so is with a colonoscope in the hands of a highly qualified digestive disease specialist. Colonoscopy is one of the best tools healthcare professionals have to detect and remove polyps before they turn into cancer, find cancer early if present, or identify other problems in the colon or rectum. To see what the colon looks like, see the "Explaining What the Colon Does" section later in the chapter.

Admittedly, colonoscopy isn't exactly a glamorous procedure. It may be slightly uncomfortable and embarrassing, but the fact remains, colonoscopy is the gold standard for preventing or catching problems in the colon and rectum.

Checking the doc's credentials

Generally the doctor who performs your colonoscopy is a *gastroenterologist,* a doctor who specializes in the digestive system and its disorders. Physicians, including gastroenterologists or surgeons, who receive specialized training in performing colonoscopies are best suited to perform the procedure.

Make sure that your colonoscopy will be done by an experienced digestive disease specialist who is interested in constant improvement in the quality of colonoscopy that he or she provides. Working with a healthcare professional who is experienced in conducting colonoscopies will increase the likelihood that your exam will be as accurate and thorough as possible.

Realizing the need

The two most common reasons to have a colonoscopy are to investigate symptoms that you may be experiencing (called a *diagnostic colonoscopy*) or for colorectal cancer screening (called *screening colonoscopy*). A colonoscopy is one of the most comprehensive methods to evaluate abnormalities within the colon, including cancer, inflammation, bleeding, and polyps, which are the precursor to *colorectal cancer.*

Colorectal cancer refers to colon and rectal cancer; although the term isn't technically synonymous with colon cancer, a lot of lay people do just say "colon cancer." (Turn to the next chapter for more info.)

The most common reasons a doctor recommends a colonoscopy other than for routine cancer screening include:

- ✔ To diagnose inflammatory bowel disease (IBD) like Crohn's disease and ulcerative colitis

- ✔ To investigate a change in bowel habits, rectal bleeding or low blood count, unexplained abdominal pain, or weight loss

Recognizing when to get one

Everyone at or over the age of 50, without any risk factors for polyps and cancer, should have a screening colonoscopy. If the exam turns out to be normal, national guidelines suggest having your next exam in ten years. Fifty is the age when people are at an increased risk for starting to develop precancerous colon polyps that can lead to colon cancer. So if you're 50 or older, schedule your screening colonoscopy now.

If you have risk factors for colon cancer — I talk about risk factors in depth in Chapter 2 — your doctor may recommend earlier and more frequent colonoscopies.

Why do people avoid getting a screening colonoscopy?

Despite the importance of colon cancer screening, people are still reluctant to get a colonoscopy. Some of the reasons people give most frequently for not getting screened include:

🖊 **They have no symptoms.** The fact is, you may not experience symptoms of colon polyps or cancer until the disease has advanced. It's always better to remove polyps before they turn into cancer or to catch colon cancer early when it's very treatable.

🖊 **They have concerns about safety.** One thing I hope you take away from this book is that colonoscopy is a common and generally safe procedure, although nothing is without risk, and colonoscopy is no different.

🖊 **They're embarrassed by the procedure.** Your privacy is of the utmost concern to your physician, their staff, and their facility. Plus, the joy in knowing you are taking a positive step in caring for your health should outweigh the potential embarrassment anticipated.

🖊 **The bowel prep is a bummer.** This statement is fairly accurate. But, if you talk to your doctor about your concerns, medical condition, medical history, and current medication use, including over-the-counter medications, your doctor may be able to pick a bowel prep that is appropriate for you. Follow all of the directions. Stay well hydrated. Chances are you can make the bowel prep process much less of a bummer.

🖊 **It's going to hurt.** Sure, the procedure may involve modest discomfort, but that's why your physician uses a moderate anesthesia called *conscious sedation*. Many people sleep through the exam and some never even remember having the colonoscopy.

🖊 **The doctor hasn't recommended it.** Believe it or not, considering the importance of screening and the ability to curb colorectal cancer, many doctors still don't make a point of recommending the procedure. If your doctor hasn't had the discussion with you by the time you're 50, start the conversation yourself.

Symptoms of colon cancer may not appear until the disease is advanced, so a screening colonoscopy when you don't have symptoms is your best chance for early detection. Polyps often don't cause any symptoms. Removing them before they turn to cancer is the best way to prevent it from developing.

Understanding Some of the Risks and Benefits

Just like other semi-invasive healthcare procedures and examinations, there are risks associated with colonoscopy and preparation for colonoscopy. The good thing is that if your health and medication (both prescription and over-the-counter) information is thoroughly discussed with and reviewed by your doctor, in most people the benefits outweigh the risks.

Potential risks of colonoscopy may include bleeding, infection, intestinal *perforation* (poking a hole in the colon), missing polyps or cancer, and adverse reactions associated with colonoscopy preps or sedatives. Many of these risks rarely occur and are even less common with a colonoscopy that doesn't involve polyp removal. You can reduce risks by ensuring that the doctor that performs the procedure is an experienced gastroenterologist or surgeon. Another great way to reduce procedural risk and increase the detection of polyps is to arrive at your procedure with a clean colon. This can be done by following your healthcare provider's directions for bowel preparation. (For more on this topic, see Chapter 3.)

The most common adverse events associated with colonoscopy preps include bloating, nausea, abdominal pain, and vomiting. Other, more serious risks have occurred as well. You'll find further information about the risks and adverse events associated with the prep for a colonoscopy in the literature regarding the preps supplied by their manufacturers and from your pharmacy. As certain medications and medical conditions may affect these events, you should fully discuss these, as well as your prep, and how to properly take it with your doctor. (For more on this topic, see Chapter 4.)

Figuring Out the Costs

The costs associated with a colonoscopy vary greatly depending on where you live, where you have the procedure done, the medicines you're given, and whether the doctor needs to do any additional procedures, such as a biopsy or polyp removal. There's no way to provide a specific cost without knowing these factors.

Insurance coverage varies widely as well. A lot of the cost, if not all, may be covered by your insurance company. Insurance will cover the procedure if you have a symptom, and more often than not it will cover a screening colonoscopy as well. Talk to your insurance carrier about which costs are and aren't covered so that you're not surprised when you receive your bill.

Check the following list for helpful info if you get benefits through Medicare or Medicaid:

- ✔ **Medicare** coverage for a colonoscopy is the same in every state. For information on what you have to pay, you can go to the Medicare Web site at `www.medicare.gov/coverage/Home.asp`. You enter the state you live in and the procedure you want to know about and get the information you need. You can also call 1-800-MEDICARE (1-800-633-4227) toll free.

- ✔ **Medicaid** isn't so simple because coverage varies by state. But you can find a lot of information at the following Web site: `www.cms.hhs.gov/home/medicaid.asp?`.

If you're uninsured, talk to your healthcare facility to discuss costs and payment options.

Additional Colorectal Cancer Screening Methods

Currently, a colonoscopy is the most comprehensive method for the detection and removal of colon polyps or for the early detection of cancer.

Although a variety of screening methods other than colonoscopy are available and have been endorsed by the American College of Gastroenterology and the U.S. Multi-Society Task Force on Colorectal Cancer, they all have advantages and disadvantages. Most individuals should choose the option that is most suitable for them. The following list includes the available methods your healthcare provider may recommend for colorectal cancer screening:

✔ **Virtual colonoscopy:** The technical name for a virtual colonoscopy is *computerized tomographic (CT) colonography* — a radiological procedure using a CT scan. Like a conventional colonoscopy, the virtual colonoscopy requires you to down a colon prep the day before the procedure to clean waste from the colon and to drink other liquids to tag the stool if any remains present in the colon at the time of the exam.

During a virtual colonoscopy, a thin tube is inserted into the rectum to inflate the colon with air. The patient lies on her stomach and then on her back inside the large CT scan imaging machine while X-rays are taken. The machine then produces a computer-generated view of the colon.

This procedure is recommended to be conducted every five years. Currently, virtual colonoscopy isn't covered by Medicare and some insurance companies. Small polyps aren't reliably detected by virtual colonoscopy, and the procedure doesn't allow the physician to perform biopsies or remove growths. If polyps or other abnormalities are detected, a colonoscopy is required to confirm the findings and remove the polyps or sample the abnormality.

✔ **Sigmoidoscopy:** This ten minute examination is similar to a colonoscopy, except the scope the doctor uses is shorter than a colonoscope and only allows a view of the lower quarter or third of the colon. It is often done without sedation after cleansing with an enema. Because the procedure doesn't allow an examination of the entire colon, it's often coupled with annual fecal occult blood testing. If a polyp is found during a sigmoidoscopy, a full colonoscopy is recommended to remove the polyp and inspect the rest of the colon. Like virtual colonoscopy, a sigmoidoscopy should be conducted every five years.

✔ **Fecal occult blood test or fecal immunochemical test (FIT):** One of the symptoms of large polyps or colon cancer is bleeding. Blood loss into the colon may be slow and chronic and not visible to the naked eye. A stool test can be performed to detect occult blood loss. To perform a fecal occult (*occult* in this context means "hidden") blood test, the healthcare provider gives you a test kit to collect samples at home. You return the samples to the healthcare provider or lab, and the sample is then tested for blood.

This fecal occult blood test should be performed yearly after you turn 50. If blood is detected, a colonoscopy is recommended to determine the cause of the bleeding. Other conditions that can cause blood in the stool include hemorrhoids, anal fissures, colon polyps, peptic ulcers, ulcerative colitis, gastroesophageal reflux disease (GERD), Crohn's disease, and damage to the intestinal tract from the use of aspirin or other nonsteroidal anti-inflammatory drugs (NSAIDs). The accuracy of FIT to detect bleeding from only the colon is higher than other methods because FIT doesn't detect upper gastrointestinal sources of blood loss.

✓ **Double contrast barium enema (DCBE):** This is an X-ray test that is done in a somewhat similar fashion to the virtual colonoscopy and should also be conducted every five years. After a thorough bowel prep, barium is put into the colon and rectum using an *enema* (a tube inserted into the rectum). The liquid barium enables a healthcare provider to see a detailed outline of the colon and rectum in an X-ray. Air is pumped in, and multiple X-rays are taken to show the outline of the colon and rectum at different angles. From the outlines, a healthcare provider may be able to detect the presence of polyps.

This screening method hasn't been shown to be reliable for the detection of polyps. When polyps are found, a colonoscopy is normally performed to confirm the results.

✓ **Fecal DNA testing:** Fecal DNA is another newly endorsed colon cancer screening method. There is no consensus on the interval at which this stool test is to be performed. Basically, a stool sample is collected and sent to a specialized lab to search for genetic mutations that can arise in large colon polyps and colon cancer. Unfortunately, the first version of fecal DNA testing only detected 50 percent of colon cancers and upgraded versions have not been studied in large screening populations yet.

So, there are several other methods that have been recommended as options for colon cancer screening, but all lead to colonoscopy if abnormalities are detected. Colonoscopy is the only exam that allows a full examination of the colon and rectum with the ability to diagnose colorectal cancer, and prevent it by removing precancerous polyps.

Explaining What the Colon Does

The *colon* is part of the large intestine, also called the *bowel*. In fact, the colon is the final 6-foot-long segment of your digestive tract. The colon is where digested food waste and bacteria are formed into solid stool. Figure 1-1 shows the digestive system.

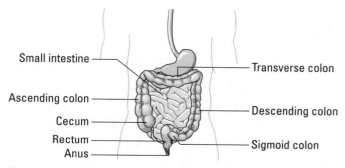

Small intestine

Ascending colon

Cecum

Rectum

Anus

Transverse colon

Descending colon

Sigmoid colon

Figure 1-1: The path food takes through your body.

To get a better feel of the big picture, consider what happens when you eat an apple: After you chew and swallow the apple, it travels down your esophagus to your stomach where it's broken down into smaller pieces by the churning action of the stomach. What's left of your apple moves from your stomach to your small intestine. The small intestine secretes fluid and digestive enzymes and absorbs nutrients from your apple. By this point, the apple no longer resembles what you ate — it may resemble applesauce, but not even that very much. The remains of your former apple move from the small intestine into the large intestine as mostly liquid. The colon removes excess water from the intestinal contents until a solid movement is formed. Bowel movements reach the left side of the colon where they are stored and can leave the body when socially acceptable.

Chapter 2

Looking at Colorectal Cancer

* *

* *

*C*olorectal cancer (CRC), which encompasses both colon and rectal cancer, refers to cancer that occurs anywhere in the large intestine, including the rectum.

According to the American Cancer Society, more than 146,000 new cases of CRC will be diagnosed in the United States this year alone — resulting in more than 49,000 deaths. That makes CRC the second leading cause of cancer-related death in the United States. Yet, colorectal cancer can be preventable through screening and removal of polyps.

Early detection of colorectal cancer leads to more successful treatment. In fact, more than 90 percent of people diagnosed when the cancer is early stage, confined to the colon or rectum, survive more than five years.

How Colon Cancer Develops

CRC usually begins as an abnormal tissue growth called a *polyp*. There are many different types of colorectal polyps, and most never turn into cancer. Adenomatous polyps are the precancerous polyps that can lead to colon cancer. It is believed to take about ten years for an adenoma to develop into a cancer. Since it is difficult to tell the underlying nature of a polyp at the time of colonoscopy, it is recommended that all polyps be removed and sent to the lab for an analysis. The removal of polyps may prevent cancer from developing from them.

Polyps are relatively common. In fact, 50 percent of people older than 60 years of age have polyps. Up to 2 percent of polyps eventually develop into cancer. Although this percentage may not be alarming, routine colon cancer screening can catch polyps early and may actually prevent cancer from occurring.

If undetected, some polyps can become cancerous over the course of several years, and, if untreated, colon cancer can spread to other parts of the body.

During a colonoscopy, your doctor spends the majority of the examination looking for changes to the normal landscape of the colon lining and removing anything that looks suspicious, like polyps. Polyps may be slightly raised (sessile), look like they are on a stalk like broccoli (pedunculated), or may be flat where they are no higher than 2.5 millimeters in height. Figure 2-1 shows the different types of colon polyps.

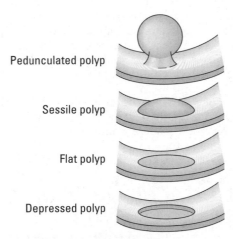

Pedunculated polyp

Sessile polyp

Flat polyp

Depressed polyp

Figure 2-1: Types of polyps.

Flat polyps may be more difficult to detect than sessile or pedunculated polyps (refer to Figure 2-1). Ensuring a very clean colon with an optimal bowel preparation prior to a colonoscopy is crucial in giving the doctor a better shot at being able to detect polyps. (The prep process is explained in Chapter 4.)

A colonoscopy can help find and remove colon polyps before they become cancerous. The aim of screening is to identify precancerous polyps or cancer in its early stage when it is curable. Colonoscopies can actually prevent cancer from developing because polyps are removed during the procedure.

Identifying the Stages

As with any cancer, colon cancer has stages that describe the extent of the cancer in the body.

What stage colon cancer is in depends on how far the cancer has grown into the walls of the intestine and beyond. Staging is based on the results of a physical exam, biopsies, and imaging tests.

The stage is essential in determining prognosis and treatment options. The earlier cancer is diagnosed, staged, and treated, the better the prospects for survival.

Colon cancer is generally staged on a scale from 0 to IV. Stage 0 is cancer in its earliest stages, when it has yet to grow beyond the inner lining of the colon. Stages I and II refer to larger cancers that have grown more deeply into, or possibly all the way through, the colon. Survival is very likely for stage I (91 percent) and stage II (80 percent) cancer. Stage III refers to cancer that has spread to lymph nodes, and the survival rate at this stage is 65 percent. Stage IV cancer has spread to other organs and is generally incurable. Stage IV survival rate is only around 10 percent.

Listing Risk Factors

Both inherited and lifestyle factors appear to play a part in the development of colon polyps and colon cancer.

Although the majority of people who develop polyps and cancer don't have any obvious risk factors, certain things are known to put you at a higher risk of developing colon cancer. I talk about each in the following sections. If you have risk factors for colon cancer, it is likely that you may require a colonoscopy at a younger age or a shorter interval between exams.

Although genetic factors may contribute to your risk for colon cancer, diet and other lifestyle factors may also impact whether you develop the disease. Still, 75 percent of all colon cancer cases occur in people with no known risk factors. This emphasizes the importance of routine colon cancer screening.

Race

African Americans have a higher risk and death rate from colon cancer than any other ethnic group. The exact reason isn't known. African Americans should begin screening colonoscopy at the age of 45 rather than the age of 50.

Age

Yes, 50 is still fabulous. It's also the age at which you need to schedule your first colonoscopy if you haven't had one already. You're more likely to start developing adenomatous polyps that can lead to colon cancer after 50 than you are before that age. A lot of things start developing after you turn 50, but while you can ignore that little paunch or those fine laugh lines, you can't ignore the possibility of colon cancer.

Although colon cancer can strike at any age, 91 percent of new cases are in people older than 50 years.

Personal or family history of adenomatous polyps and CRC

If you or an immediate family member (parent, sibling, or child) has a history of precancerous colon polyps or colon cancer, you are at a two- to threefold increased risk of getting adenomatous polyps or colon cancer. Very rarely, colon cancer can be caused by an inherited syndrome such as *hereditary nonpolyposis colorectal cancer (HNPCC)* or *familial adenomatous polyposis (FAP)*. People with these inherited syndromes have a high likelihood to develop colon cancer during their lives.

Find out as much as you can about the details of a family member's colonoscopy findings, such as how old they were when they were diagnosed, the type, size, and how numerous their polyps were, and any information about the cancer when it was diagnosed.

A personal history of inflammatory bowel disease

Inflammatory bowel disease (IBD) refers to a group of inflammatory conditions of the intestines. Ulcerative colitis and Crohn's disease are the most common forms of IBD. IBD shouldn't be confused with irritable bowel syndrome (IBS), which doesn't cause inflammation and isn't associated with colon cancer (see the nearby sidebar for a discussion of both).

A personal history of Crohn's or ulcerative colitis puts you at higher risk for developing colon cancer. The risk is dependant on the length of the colon that is affected and the length of time since the diagnosis has been made.

If you have a personal or family history of colon polyps or cancer, talk to your healthcare provider about when you need to schedule a colonoscopy.

Telling the difference between IBD and IBS

Colon cancer isn't the only disease to which the colon and intestines are subject. IBD (inflammatory bowel disease) and IBS (irritable bowel syndrome) are two often-confused conditions of the intestinal tract. Although they share some common symptoms, IBD — most commonly in the form of Crohn's disease or ulcerative colitis — may lead to bleeding, inflammation, and cancer, and IBS doesn't.

IBS

Irritable bowel syndrome (IBS) commonly causes cramping, abdominal pain, bloating, gas, diarrhea, and constipation. Despite these uncomfortable, sometimes severe signs and symptoms, IBS doesn't cause permanent damage to your colon.

Like ulcerative colitis and Crohn's disease, IBS is often not medically curable, although medication is used to treat symptoms. Thankfully it doesn't cause intestinal inflammation, bleeding, require surgery, or increase your risk of colorectal cancer.

IBD

Inflammatory bowel disease (IBD) is characterized by symptoms similar to those of IBS, but differs in that it is a collection of disorders characterized by chronic inflammation of the colon lining. The two most common forms of IBD are ulcerative colitis and Crohn's disease. Although the diseases have some features in common, there are some important differences:

- ✔ **Ulcerative colitis (UC):** In UC, the inner lining *(mucosa)* of the large intestine becomes inflamed — meaning the lining of the intestinal wall reddens and swells, often developing sores *(ulcers)*, which can bleed. Ulcerative colitis always affects the rectum but may also involve higher parts of the colon. Diarrhea, mucus, and blood often appear in the feces if the lining of the colon is inflamed. Healthcare practitioners usually prescribe a medication to help reduce the inflammation, but more severe cases may call for surgery to remove all or part of the colon.

- ✔ **Crohn's disease:** Crohn's disease may affect the colon or other areas of the digestive tract. When inflammation in the intestines due to Crohn's disease occurs, diarrhea, abdominal pain, fever, loss of appetite, and weight loss may occur. Symptoms may range from mild to severe.

Crohn's disease generally tends to involve the entire bowel wall, whereas ulcerative colitis affects only the lining of the bowel. Crohn's is most common in the final section of the small intestine *(terminal ileum)* and parts of the large intestine, but it can affect any part of the digestive tract from the mouth to the anus.

Doctors don't know what causes IBD, and treatments include medications, diet changes, and, when necessary, surgery. In addition, patients are often encouraged to incorporate lifestyle changes into their daily activities.

Lifestyle factors

Your mother's colon cancer is a risk factor you can't avoid, but you can change your own unhealthy behavior.

- ✔ **Poor diet:** A diet high in fat (including red meat, fried foods, and high-fat dairy products) and low in fruits, grains, and vegetables may increase the risk of colon cancer.

- ✔ **Smoking:** Maybe the strongest associated risk factor, smoking may double the risk of developing colon cancer.

- ✔ **Excess alcohol use:** In addition to potentially damaging your liver, pancreas, cardiovascular system, and more, excessive alcohol use increases the risk of developing CRC.

- ✔ **Sedentary lifestyle:** Add lowering CRC risk to the list of benefits associated with an active lifestyle.

- ✔ **Obesity:** Like smoking, obesity may increase the risk up to twofold.

Recognizing the Symptoms

Symptoms of colon cancer may vary from person to person, but it's important to understand that there may be no signs at all. Colon cancer usually begins as a polyp in the colon. In general, a polyp doesn't cause any initial symptoms, but over time, it may grow and eventually become cancerous.

Finding online colon cancer resources

The Internet offers a variety of free resources where you can get information on colon cancer and ways to reduce your risks. Many of the Web sites in the following list are searchable and all are packed with helpful facts and figures to help inform and support people affected by colorectal cancer:

✔ American Cancer Society: www. cancer.org

✔ American College of Gastroenterology: www.acg. gi.org

✔ American Gastroenterological Association: www.gastro. org

✔ American Society for Gastrointestinal Endoscopy: www.asge.org

✔ American Society of Colon and Rectal Surgeons: www. fascrs.org

✔ Center for Disease Control and Prevention: www.cdc.gov

✔ Cleveland Clinic: www.cleveland clinic.org/score

✔ Colon Cancer Alliance: www. ccalliance.org

✔ National Cancer Institute: http://seer.cancer. gov

By the time a person begins experiencing symptoms associated with colon cancer, the polyp may have turned cancerous.

If you experience the symptoms in the following list, you don't necessarily have colon cancer; they're simply common symptoms that may also occur with colon cancer:

✔ Abdominal pain

✔ Anemia

✔ Blood in the stool

✔ Change in bowel habits (diarrhea, constipation, or other)

✔ Rectal bleeding or low blood count

✔ Weakness

✔ Weight loss

If you experience any of these signs, please discuss them with your healthcare provider immediately. Your healthcare provider can determine your level of risk and proceed with the proper course of action.

If you've reached 50, getting a colonoscopy is important even when you have no symptoms.

Preventing Colon Cancer

Colon cancer can be prevented by removing precancerous polyps or abnormal growths in the colon before they develop into invasive cancer. This is done routinely during a colonoscopy.

Medical professionals continue to discover more about colon cancer and the factors that influence its development. As knowledge increases, more effective screening tools are developed to help detect the disease in its early stages. The state-of-the-art prevention tool is a colonoscopy.

Estimates show that with simple lifestyle changes and widespread routine screening, nearly 30,000 lives in the United States could be saved each year.

However, despite the fact that screening methods, including colonoscopy, are very effective, colon cancer screening remains underused and lags far behind screening for breast and cervical cancers.

According to the Centers for Disease Control and Prevention, 60 percent of deaths from colorectal cancer could be prevented if everyone age 50 and older were screened appropriately, according to their risk factors.

The fact is, colon cancer is often preventable when the early warning signs are detected through routine screening (colonoscopy). If colon cancer does occur, it's treated more successfully when caught early. (See the sidebar "Facing the stats about colon cancer" for more information.)

Facing the stats about colon cancer

Simple lifestyle changes and widespread routine screening could prevent more than half of all instances of colon cancer. In theory, this could prevent 74,000 cases of colon cancer and nearly 25,000 deaths per year in the United States.

In fact, more than 90 percent of people diagnosed when the cancer is confined to the colon or rectum survive more than five years. Still, less than 50 percent of Americans aged 50 and older are routinely screened.

These figures can serve as inspiration to get the word out. Encourage people you know to get screened for colon cancer as soon as they can.

Once they reach the age of 50, people should get a colonoscopy once every 10 years, unless at higher risk. The people at greatest risk are those with a personal or family history of colon polyps or cancer, or a personal history of Crohn's or ulcerative colitis. Individuals with lifestyle risk factors such as smoking, or being overweight or obese may be recommended by their physician to have a shortened screening interval.

Don't wait for symptoms to occur: Get screened when you're supposed to get screened.

Chapter 3

Planning for Your Colonoscopy

· ·

In This Chapter

▶ Making a plan for safety and accuracy

▶ Knowing what to do

▶ Stocking up

· ·

Getting ready for your colonoscopy starts with having a plan and knowing your part in it. Being able to plan ahead of time can relieve some of the anxiety.

In this chapter, I offer a general plan to help you go into your colonoscopy informed.

Making a Plan with Your Doctor

Having a frank and honest relationship with your healthcare providers generally leads to better health for you. After your healthcare team tells you that you need a colonoscopy, ask what the procedure is, who will be performing it, and what you need to do before and after the procedure. A detailed conversation now can make for a clear mind and a clear colon later, which is what you need for accurate screening results.

The doctor or nurse will talk with you about the procedure, and tell you how to prepare your colon before the colonoscopy. (I go through the bowel-prep process in Chapter 4.) Make sure and discuss your medical history and conditions, as well as the medications you are taking, with your doctor — this information needs to be provided to your doctor so he or she can determine the bowel prep that is best for you. You will be given instructions that will explain what you should and should not do in preparation for the colonoscopy. Make sure that you understand and follow all of those instructions.

Don't be afraid to ask questions. You want to prepare properly to give your doctor the best chance of getting an optimal view of your colon.

Considering Drugs, Allergies, and Other Conditions

When you get scheduled for your colonoscopy, you must be prepared to think about how fasting, dehydration, and potential removal of pieces and parts of your colon may affect your underlying medical conditions and medications. Discuss these issues with your healthcare providers.

Review the instructions about the colonoscopy process at least two weeks ahead of time to ensure that you know what to do with your diet and medications, especially if you have diabetes, hypertension, heart, kidney, or vascular problems, require blood thinners, or have other serious medical problems. Understand that even over-the-counter medications, including herbal supplements and vitamins, can impact the potential risk of colonoscopy.

All of these issues need to be fully discussed with your doctor and thought about well ahead of the colonoscopy. Only under your prescribing physician's recommendations should you withhold or change the dose of certain medications and supplements, including blood thinners, anti-platelet agents, aspirin and other anti-inflammatories, hypertension medications, and diabetes medications.

Making Arrangements for the Day of Your Colonoscopy

Part of planning for your colonoscopy entails getting all the details down. While the colonoscopy itself is just a short part of one day, you need to take care of certain things ahead of time. I cover those essentials in the following sections.

Read through the complete instructions and information concerning your colonoscopy and the bowel prep selected by your doctors at least two weeks before your colonoscopy. Make sure you fully understand all such information and instructions before you start your bowel preparation. Contact your healthcare providers if you have any concerns or questions. Also advise your providers if there has been any change in your health status or medications (prescription or over-the-counter) in the time between your last visit and your colonoscopy.

Arrange for time off work

Take the entire day of the procedure off work. You'll most likely be sedated, so you'll be groggy and your reaction time slower. When you consider the stress your body endures completing the bowel prep and undergoing the colonoscopy itself, you really are better off taking the day off and resting at home after the examination — you've earned it!

Schedule a ride

If you're planning to have sedation at the time of your colonoscopy (as the overwhelming majority of individuals who undergo colonoscopy do), you will be required to have someone accompany you and drive you from the colonoscopy facility. The facility rules (and liability laws) don't allow you to leave or drive yourself home, and you can't even take any transportation by yourself. Ideally, you should have someone who can spend the rest of the day with you at home as well.

It may be an inconvenience, but for your own safety you need a friend or family member there with you in order to be discharged.

Get your prescription

Several different types of bowel preps are currently available, so be sure to ask your healthcare provider about the various options, the risks and benefits of each, and which prep may be most appropriate for you. When your healthcare provider settles on a prep for you, discuss how it works, how you're supposed to take it, and any other questions you have about the process.

Get to the pharmacy as soon possible after your colonoscopy is scheduled to pick up your bowel preparation (I'll discuss bowel preps at greater length in Chapter 4). You should review and understand all the instructions and information provided with your medication, and you should talk with your doctor if you have any questions or concerns. Be sure that the pharmacy has the prescription you expect, you understand the information and instructions concerning the prescription, and there is no surprise with the cost.

Stock up on supplies

After you start taking the colonoscopy prep medication, you won't want to leave the house (the next chapter explains why, but you've probably gathered that you won't want to be far from a bathroom). So stock up on what you need before you ever begin taking the medication. While you're at the pharmacy, you can also check out the magazine section, hard candies, and other supplies that you may want during the preparation process!

Go over your prep instructions and ensure you fully understand how to take the prep and have everything you need to complete the prepping process. The prep process may include some or all of the following items:

- ✔ A variety of clear liquids — check out the "Just what is a clear liquid?" sidebar for choices
- ✔ Soft toilet paper
- ✔ Wet wipes
- ✔ Lotions/creams to ease anal irritation
- ✔ Reading materials, movies, and other ways to help pass the time

Plan your "last meal"

After you start the prepping process, you can't eat solid food until after your colonoscopy, so many people like to celebrate this step toward managing their health by either cooking a special meal or making reservations at a nice restaurant.

Just what is a clear liquid?

As a category, *clear liquids* is broader than you might think. It's more than just water and lemon-lime soda. The variety of liquids that qualify as clear may surprise you; they usually include the following:

- Water (the original clear liquid)

- Chicken or beef bouillon/broth (low sodium)

- Flavored drink mix (lemonade, lime, orange flavors only)

- Frozen ice pops or Italian ice (no ice cream, sherbets, or fruit bars)

- Fruit juices so long as they're strained, without pulp (apple, white grape, white cranberry, orange, and lemonade, for example)

- Gelatin (lemon, lime, or orange only; no fruit or toppings)

- Hard candies, as long as they're not red or purple

- Soft drinks (orange, ginger ale, cola, and lemon-lime soda for example)

- Tea or coffee (no milk or non-dairy creamer)

Note: Don't drink or eat anything colored red or purple and skip alcoholic beverages while you prep.

Check with your doctor's office for a list of acceptable clear liquids.

Changing Your Diet for a Bit

Depending on your doctor's instructions, you will be expected to stop eating solid foods and drink only clear fluids for up to a day or two before the procedure to minimize the production of solid waste in your colon and rectum.

You'll be told to drink a lot of liquids before, during, and after your bowel preparation to keep you hydrated. Drinking a lot probably won't be a problem because in the process of cleaning out your colon, you lose a lot of fluid and will likely be thirsty. But even if you don't feel especially thirsty, keep drinking. I can't stress enough how important it is that you drink plenty of water or other acceptable liquids to stay hydrated. You should contact your doctor if you have any difficulties or problems with your bowel preparation.

You'll also get a list of what you can and can't eat and drink. You're generally safe with *clear liquids* — a concept I explain from a colonoscopy perspective in the nearby sidebar, "Just what is a clear liquid?"

Even though gin, vodka, and white wine are clear liquids, any alcoholic beverage is a no-no for the day or two prior to your colonoscopy — it's not a dinner party, after all. Alcohol increases the likelihood of dehydration, which is no fun whatsoever. Being dehydrated is much more than just feeling "parched." Dehydration will rock your world in a bad way. It makes you feel *really* sick, and combine that with frequent trips to the toilet and you have perfect conditions for a terrible day. Definitely call your doctor if you feel as though you might be dehydrated — it is a serious situation. And keep the chardonnay chilled until after your colonoscopy is complete and you're feeling back to normal.

Don't drink or eat anything colored red or purple. Dark coloring in your colon can lead to inaccuracies during the colonoscopy.

Setting Out a Colonoscopy Timetable

Typically, you start preparing for a colonoscopy two weeks before the actual event. Figure 3-1 shows a typical timeline of what to do when.

The information in the table is a generalized plan, which your doctor may alter according to your unique needs. Follow the specific plan your doctor provides for you and contact him or her if you have any doubts, questions, or concerns.

Two Weeks Before	A Week or More Before	Three Days Before	One Day Before	The Day of	During the Exam	After the Exam
Pick up the prep	Get time off of work	Know and follow the instructions for your prep medication	Follow instructions for prep medication	If splitting the dose, see instructions for completing your bowel prep as provided by your doctor	Follow doctor's directions — this part is pretty much out of your hands!	Drink plenty of clear liquids and stay near a toilet
Read prep instructions	Schedule transportation to and from procedure	Low residue diet	Clear liquid diet			Follow doctor's directions, and call your doctor if you experience any other conditions or problems after your colonoscopy is completed
			Drink plenty of clear liquids	Drink plenty of clear liquids, but not anything after the specified time		
Contact your doctor if there are any changes in your medical condition or medications (prescription or over-the-counter)	Adjust medications according to doctor's orders		Stay near a toilet	Stay near a toilet		Return to your normal diet unless otherwise instructed by your doctor
	Stock up on necessities including clear liquids, toilet paper, wet wipes, lotion		Call your doctor if you are unable to finish your prep or if you have any questions or concerns	Arrive at the facility at the designated time		

Figure 3-1: Colonoscopy timetable.

Chapter 4

Explaining the Bowel Prep Process

● ●

In This Chapter

▶ Prepping the colon cleans the colon

▶ Looking at your prep options

▶ Communicating with your doctor

▶ Hydrating is essential

▶ Following all instructions and directions

● ●

*I*f you ask anyone who's gone through a colonoscopy, they'll probably tell you that the procedure is relatively easy and that the preparation was the hard part. It's true, preparing for a colonoscopy certainly isn't pleasant, but understanding the importance should help you keep a positive outlook.

Providing information about your health to your doctor, understanding the information about your bowel prep, and following all instructions concerning your bowel prep are your primary responsibilities throughout the entire colonoscopy process. Don't wait until the day before the procedure to read the prep instructions, and don't wait to talk with your doctor about your health and your medications. There are steps you may have to take seven to ten days prior to your colonoscopy (for a detailed timetable, see Chapter 3). How well you clean out your colon determines how well your doctor can see the colon lining and detect potential problems.

Understanding the Process

Completing the bowel preparation solution is the greatest challenge to undergoing colonoscopy. They simply don't taste very good, but prep manufacturers have taken steps to make the preps more tolerable. Granted, it still isn't something you'd choose to do as a pastime, but cleaning the colon is an absolutely critical part of an effective procedure.

A *bowel prep* (also called *colon prep* or *colonoscopy prep*) is a prescription medicine your doctor gives you to prepare your bowel for inspection during a colonoscopy. There are different types of bowel preps. You must provide your doctor with information concerning your medical history and conditions, as well as information concerning your medications, so he or she can prescribe the bowel prep that is appropriate for you. The objective of a bowel prep is to remove all solid waste from the digestive tract. Your colon needs to be completely empty of all waste (stool) before your colonoscopy so that your doctor can actually see your colon walls. The *colonoscope* — the long, thin tool with a camera attached that travels through your colon during a colonoscopy — can't see through solids.

The bowel prep medicine quickly eliminates solid waste from the digestive tract — another way of saying it causes diarrhea. So stay near a toilet while you're completing the prep process.

Your doctor will be looking for any colorectal abnormalities, but especially for polyps and cancer. These can be tiny, so even the smallest amount of waste could potentially disguise something important. Therefore, your colon must be thoroughly cleansed before the exam to give your doctor the best chance for a thorough examination.

 Don't eat during the prep process. Eating during the bowel prep process creates fecal material that collects in your colon and makes it difficult for your doctor to inspect the lining.

Staying hydrated

A huge component of how well you tolerate the prep process has to do with how well hydrated you stay. The prepping process pulls a lot of water from your body, so you need to replace that water by drinking clear liquids. Hydration is essential for an effective and safe colonoscopy prep.

Colon cleansing causes the body to lose fluids quickly, which can lead to dehydration regardless of the specific prep that you take. Even mild dehydration will give you a dull, sick feeling and if you feel bad, you won't be motivated to complete your prep.

If you become dehydrated, you may experience extreme thirst, dizziness, headaches, chill, and nausea. If you have ever experienced these symptoms you know that drinking more bowel prep is probably not in your top ten list of things you would like to do next. In fact, calling your doctor should be the first thing you do if you become dehydrated.

To stay hydrated, you need to replace the fluids you're losing, so drink plenty of clear liquids. It's also important to stay hydrated after your procedure, so continue drinking liquids. Many of the bowel preps' dosing regimens help with proper hydration during colonoscopy preparation, so follow your doctor's bowel prep instructions carefully. Contact your doctor if you have any questions or concerns regarding your bowel prep, the instructions regarding your bowel prep, or you have any difficulty when taking your bowel prep.

Drink plenty of clear liquids before, during, and after the colon-prep process. A clear liquid is any beverage you can see through that doesn't contain red or purple colors or pulp. See Chapter 3 for a comprehensive list of acceptable clear liquids.

Following the Instructions

Most people have heard the stories of having to drink a gallon of foul-tasting liquid to prep for their colonoscopy. The fact is, there are choices when it comes to bowel preps. They don't all involve a full gallon of liquid, and some even incorporate your choice of clear liquid to supplement the active ingredient. Preps vary in the active ingredient they use, how they taste, how much liquid is involved, and in how they're dosed. The manufacturers have worked over the years to develop prep options that are more tolerable.

Different bowel preps flush out the colon using different methods. Talk to your doctor about the various choices and which prep may be appropriate for you, as your doctor considers many factors in deciding which prep you should use. You need to tell your doctor about your medical history and condition, as well as the medications (both prescription and over-the-counter) you're taking, so he or she can determine the bowel prep that is best for you. Whichever prep you end up taking, remember to drink plenty of liquids, stay hydrated, and follow the instructions while you go through this process. No matter what prep you take, follow the instructions provided with the prep as well as your doctor's instructions.

Your doctor's instructions will depend on the type of prep prescribed, the time of your colonoscopy procedure, and your specific needs. The key to a successful colonoscopy is to follow your healthcare professional's bowel prep instructions.

Don't be afraid to ask questions. Bowel prep is an essential part of a successful colonoscopy, so you need to make sure that you completely understand the instructions provided concerning your bowel prep.

Splitting the Dose

Split-dosing refers to taking at least part of the prep medication on the day of the procedure — about five hours prior to the scheduled procedure time.

Clinical studies show that taking at least part of the prep on the day of the procedure can significantly improve the quality of the preparation for colonoscopy. In the past, healthcare providers had patients take all the prep medication the night before. This is an effective way to clean the colon, but leaves the potential for intestinal secretions from the small intestine to enter the right side of the large intestine in the time between the end of the prep process the evening before and the start of the colonoscopy. This right side of the large intestine is an important area because cancers commonly develop there. Flatter polyps are common in this area and can be hard to see even with a perfect bowel preparation.

Your doctor will give you instructions that he or she believes will maximize the effectiveness and safety of your bowel prep. But you can certainly discuss the pros and cons of the different bowel preps and the possibility of split-dosing with your healthcare provider.

Setting Aside Some Sitting Time

I understand that you're busy and you want to get in that last errand between prep doses. You gotta do what you gotta do. All I can say is that it's impossible to predict when the prep's effects are going to kick in. Most people experience a bowel movement within a couple hours of starting a bowel prep, but this varies from person to person. When the effects of the prep make themselves felt, you will definitely be the first to know, and you'll probably know pretty urgently. So ask yourself how important that errand really is.

Call your physician if you have any problems completing the prep or if you experience unexpected effects from the prep or no effects from the prep after several hours.

You go to the bathroom a lot — and I mean a *lot* — as the bowel prep goes to work. You want to know how many times, and I answer: as many times as it takes. I know, that's not a really precise answer, but different people have different results. If you follow all of the directions and complete your prep medication in the proper time frame, you will give your prep the best chance to work.

Stock your bathroom with plenty of entertainment — reading material, puzzle books, handheld games, a personal DVD player — and soft wipes.

I have another iffy answer for how to know when your bowel is clean: There's no sure way to know until your doctor begins the colonoscopy. Just follow your doctor's bowel prep instructions to the letter. At some point you'll notice the color of your diarrhea getting lighter, which is generally a sign that less material is being cleaned from the colon, meaning your colon is getting cleaner. That doesn't mean you should stop — finish your prep as directed by your doctor!

Tips to keep things moving smoothly

As you prepare for bowel prep, keep these tips in mind:

✔ **Talk to your doctor.** Inform your doctor about your medical history and condition, as well as the medications you are taking (including any over-the-counter medications or supplements) when discussing different bowel prep options.

✔ **Complete the prep.** A clean colon results in the most effective colonoscopy, and your prep is more likely to be thorough if you complete the entire regimen.

Your physician will provide you with detailed instructions to prepare you for your colonoscopy — follow them exactly. You don't want to have to do the prep all over again because you didn't get it right the first time.

✔ **Stay hydrated.** Being hydrated before, during, and after the prep and colonoscopy is very important.

✔ **Get comfortable and stay comfortable.** Once you start drinking the prep, be prepared to spend a lot of time on the toilet. Bring a book — or two. And to take care of your tush, use adult wet wipes or a water spray to clean off instead of toilet paper.

✔ **Enjoy some variety.** Keep plenty of clear liquids on hand to drink. Water gets boring and you need to stay hydrated.

✔ **Call your doctor with questions.** Call the doctor's office for help if you have any trouble, don't understand the prep instructions, or have any questions about the bowel prep medication prescribed for you.

The prep generally keeps working for several hours. How long depends partly on your body's ability to pass the active ingredient.

After the prep starts working, continue to drink clear fluids and finish the prep as directed by your doctor.

Recognizing the Risks of an Incomplete Prep

If you don't prep well enough, there will be fecal matter left in the colon. Your doctor may be unable to see the inside surface of your colon clearly. He or she may spend more time looking around and still not be able to see potential problems, which isn't good news for anybody.

If your colon isn't clean enough, the doctor may decide to stop the procedure and ask you to reschedule. This means you have to repeat the bowel prep process, reschedule a driver, miss another day of work, and possibly absorb the cost and risk of the second procedure. And that's not even the worst part: You may be delaying treatment of something that could be very serious.

Although the prepping process isn't exactly pleasant, doing it well can save you a lot of hassle. Read the directions thoroughly, understand and follow them, and contact your doctor if you have any questions or concerns. A good prep will mean a thorough examination.

 If you don't prep at all, your colon stays dirty and your doctor can't see anything. Follow all instructions and contact your doctor if you have any problems related to the completion of, or in connection with, your prep.

Paying Attention to Potential Problems

Cleansing your bowel over the course of a few hours doesn't make for a comfortable experience. Talk to your doctor about what are normal occurrences during the prepping process and if you have any questions as to how to properly complete the process.

Some minor side effects are common during the prep; some nausea, bloating, and abdominal distention. If you chilled the prep prior to drinking it, you could experience some shaking chills from consuming so much cold liquid in a short time period. These minor types of side effects call for holding off on the prep for a bit, then trying to restart after the symptoms pass. If you can't restart, call the doctor for recommendations. Although no fun to experience, these side effects are very common. They unfortunately go hand-in-hand with ingesting 2 to 4 liters of fluid in a short period of time. But it's a problem if these side effects become severe or continue after completing the prep.

Other side effects such as dizziness, fever, or severe headache are much less common and are probably more serious. They could indicate dehydration or allergic reaction and should result in an immediate call to the doctor. More serious side effects are possible and have been reported as well — they're discussed in the product information and Medication Guides provided by the manufacturers of the bowel preps. You should review this information when you get your prescription and contact your doctor with any questions or concerns. Listen to your body during the bowel prep process. Persistent or severe side effects shouldn't be overlooked, and it's always better to be safe than sorry. If you're worried about a potential side effect, call your doctor.

Chapter 5

Experiencing the Colonoscopy Procedure

. . . .

In This Chapter

▶ Expecting the best

▶ Zipping through the procedure itself

▶ Resting up afterward

. . . .

*W*hen it comes to the actual colonoscopy procedure, your physician's journey is beginning, while yours is almost over. You may be surprised by how quickly it goes. Maybe it's the medication they give you before the procedure. Maybe it's sleep deprivation. Maybe it's just that the actual colonoscopy procedure is a breeze, according to most people who have one. The hard part of the process, the bowel prep, is already complete.

But describing the scenery to someone who hasn't traveled the road does little to prepare them for their trip. I can only hope to calm some anxiety by answering some questions in this chapter.

Expecting Paperwork, Meds, and Feeling No Pain

Make sure to report any problems or difficulties you had during the bowel prep process when you arrive at the colo-noscopy facility. Once there, you'll probably have to sign a few forms — don't you always? You'll be shown to a private area in the pre-procedure room where you change into an examination gown — be sure to take off your underwear! A nurse will insert an IV line and review your medications, allergies, and medical history. Then you're taken to a private colonoscopy suite, where your potentially immodest hospital attire is seen only by professionals, who've seen it all before.

Your privacy and safety are of the utmost concern to your physicians, their staff, and their facility. Your colonoscopy will be conducted in a private area specially outfitted with the tools needed to complete the procedure.

The medical staff outfits you with several different devices that help monitor your vital signs during the colonoscopy — this is the routine for all colonoscopy patients.

Your doctor and healthcare team who will be assisting with the procedure will discuss your medical history, the procedure details including risks and benefits, and answer any questions you may have. Once you're comfortable that all your questions have been answered, it's time to start the procedure.

Going through the Procedure

You begin the procedure by lying on your left side on an examination table. You're given sedation through your IV and should start feeling the effects fairly quickly.

The most common method of sedation for a colonoscopy, called *conscious sedation,* puts you into a sleepy, dreamlike state to make you comfortable for the procedure. Although some patients sleep, others are conscious during the colonoscopy. You may even talk with the doctor or nurse during the procedure, but more than likely, receiving the sedative will be the last thing you remember. But even if you're not aware of it, the doctor and medical staff monitor your vital signs throughout the procedure.

Talking about the tool

A colonoscopy involves the use of a *colonoscope* — a long, thin, flexible instrument connected to a camera with a light source and video display monitor as shown in Figure 5-1.

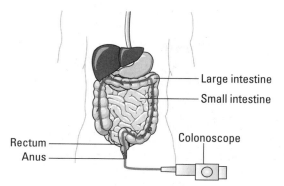

Rectum

Anus

Large intestine

Small intestine

Colonoscope

Figure 5-1: A look at how a colonoscope works.

A doctor, usually a gastroenterologist or colorectal surgeon, inserts the colonoscope into the anus, through the rectum, and into the rest of the colon until reaching the end of the colon, called the cecum. This takes about 15 minutes. The scope allows the doctor to instill and remove water, if necessary for additional cleansing, or to inflate and remove air from the large intestine for an optimal view of the colon lining. The optics of the scope transmit a video image from inside the large intestine to a computer screen. The scope is then slowly removed while the doctor carefully checks the colon lining for polyps or other abnormalities. The design of the colonoscope makes it possible to pass instruments through the channel of the scope to sample or remove tissue — often without the need for surgery.

Removing polyps and doing biopsies as needed

During the course of your colonoscopy, if your doctor sees a polyp or other growth or lesion, he or she may remove it in its entirety or a piece of it if it's too big to safely be removed with a colonoscope. The equipment used includes forceps or a snare. Take a look at Figure 5-2 to see the biopsy forceps and snare. You can see that there are multiple channels at the tip of the scope — the snare comes out of one, the forceps come out of another.

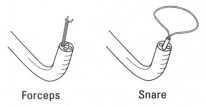

Forceps   Snare

Figure 5-2: The snare and forceps.

A *biopsy* is performed on the removed tissue, meaning the tissue is sent to a laboratory to determine the nature of the lesion.

Most colon cancer starts as noncancerous polyps. Because the underlying nature of colon polyps can't be accurately determined without biopsy, most polyps are removed during colonoscopy.

The colon doesn't feel pinching or burning sensations, so you'll be glad to know that people don't feel a polyp being removed. The colon pain receptors do feel the stretching sensation from air distension.

Tissue is removed in two general ways:

- ✔ **Polypectomy:** In order to remove a polyp, a tweezerlike instrument called *forceps* or a flexible wire loop called a *snare* can be passed through the scope to cut out the polyp. Either of these methods can be used cold or hot. Hot means with the use of cautery or heat to burn the tissue.

- ✔ **Biopsy:** In a *biopsy,* the doctor removes a small amount of tissue for the lab to examine and determine its microscopic nature. This method is used on a polyp or tumor too big to be safely removed through the scope. This helps to determine the nature of the lesion and its appropriate evaluation and treatment.

  The tissue is retrieved through the channel of the scope, or if it is too big, it is dragged out with a basket as the scope is removed from the colon.

Heading Home Afterward

The entire colonoscopy procedure usually takes less than half an hour. You arrive 30 minutes early to spend a few minutes beforehand with the paperwork, changing, IV insertion, nurse's intake form, and you spend maybe half-an-hour in the recovery room. So, generally, a couple hours after you walk into the facility, you're ready to be driven home.

The time you spend in the recovery room is dictated according to safety standards and to ensure your vital signs are acceptable for discharge. The sedative can stay in the blood for up to 24 hours and the effects of sedation can be subtle. Many people have little memory of the colonoscopy.

After you've recovered a bit, the doctor usually provides you with a copy of the procedure report, complete with pictures, and tells you what has been found. Most often, patients are told whether something of concern has been found or not and what the follow-up plan is. Often the family member or driver is at bedside when the procedure results are being discussed, as the patient may still be a little foggy from the sedation. Most providers also send a letter to the patient with the results of the biopsies and the interval for the next colonoscopy.

Because you've been sedated, you may not drive until the next day. You need to have someone accompany you from the recovery area and drive you home after the procedure. For your safety, the staff at the facility can't let you leave by yourself.

Because air is pumped into your colon during the colonoscopy and may not be completely removed, you may experience some slight discomfort and bloating for a few hours following the colonoscopy. Feel free to let the gas pass if it is present — you'll feel better. You may be embarrassed by the process, but don't worry, you will be part of the wind section in the recovery unit and it will pass, usually within 24 hours.

If you experience pain, bloating, or excessive rectal bleeding following the procedure, contact your healthcare provider as soon as possible. In addition, tell your doctor if you experience any other conditions or problems after your colonoscopy is completed.

Plan on resting for the remainder of the day, and eat lightly at first. Minor symptoms such as gas or bloating will disappear within 24 hours.

Chapter 6

Getting Back to Normal after Your Colonoscopy

*Y*ou've fasted. You've hydrated. You've prepped. You've spent quality time with your plumbing. Your doctor has gone where no one has gone before. The colonoscopy is behind you, and you can begin to get back to your normal life — just make sure you do it slowly.

Even after your colonoscopy, you have a few things to keep in mind. Discharge instructions will be provided by the personnel in the recovery room. They will give you an idea of what to expect over the course of the next 24 hours, including restrictions on any medications or activities.

Again, follow your healthcare provider's instructions for what to do after your colonoscopy and report any problems or concerns to him or her as soon as possible. This chapter has a few recommendations.

Leaving the Car Parked for the Day

Those "don't operate heavy machinery" warnings apply to you when you get home from your colonoscopy. You may feel fine, but the lingering effects of the sedation can noticeably affect your reaction time. So, keep the car and the forklift parked until the next day. You can resume your normal activities, including driving, the following day, unless your doctor told you otherwise.

Getting Back to Eating

After missing at least a couple of meals before your colonoscopy, you may feel a little hungry afterwards. You can start eating again, although you may want to choose something light to start with.

Sometimes the prepping process leaves your digestive system extra sensitive, so be gentle. Make your first meal something you can digest easily. Start slowly and build up your tolerance. If your appetite doesn't return, let your physician know.

You should be able to eat and drink like normal, unless otherwise instructed.

 Throughout the prepping process, your body lost a lot of water and some electrolytes. Drink plenty of fluids to replace those lost. However, you may be asked to avoid drinking alcohol for some period of time after the colonoscopy. Alcohol tends to dehydrate, and you need to rehydrate.

Paying Attention to Post-Procedure Symptoms

Your body isn't used to what you've gone through in the last 24 to 48 hours, with the colonoscopy and the prep process — it's not like you do this every day. Because the colon was filled with air so that the doctor could see the lining very well, you may experience some mild abdominal discomfort or bloating, both of which are perfectly normal after a colonoscopy. And, yes, you're going to have some gas. But you really shouldn't expect any significant discomfort.

Your physician's office will provide you with a detailed list of discharge instructions before you leave the recovery area. These will include lists of expected and unexpected symptoms.

You will be given phone numbers in case any symptoms develop or you have concerns. So talk with your healthcare providers before your discharge about any of your concerns or symptoms. Remember, it's always easier to deal with a problem in the early stages than it is if you let it go and let it get worse. Contact your doctor if you experience any unexpected problems or if you have any questions or concerns.

Call your doctor immediately if you experience any of the symptoms listed on your post-colonoscopy discharge sheet, which may include but are not limited to:

- ✔ Chills or fever
- ✔ Rectal bleeding (more than a tablespoon)
- ✔ Swelling or redness at your IV site
- ✔ Severe abdominal pain or bloating
- ✔ Persistent nausea or vomiting
- ✔ Extreme thirst
- ✔ Dizziness
- ✔ Headaches

Following Up on Polyps

When a polyp is removed from the colorectal lining, a small ulcer or sore remains at the removal site, which can be prone to bleeding, either immediately or within two weeks. If you had polyps removed during your colonoscopy, your doctor may make special recommendations about your use of medications, including over-the-counter medications, herbs, or supplements to minimize the risk of bleeding from the polyp removal site.

Make sure you and your doctor develop a plan for resuming any medications.

Immediately after the procedure, your doctor will be able to reassure you or advise you whether there was something serious or concerning detected on the examination, even without the results of biopsies. The majority of individuals undergoing colonoscopy get reassuring news that the exam was normal or that nothing found on the exam is life threatening. If your doctor is very concerned about something found on the exam, the biopsy sample can be rushed through the process in the lab for quicker results. Routine processing usually takes less than one week.

Waiting for results of biopsies can be unnerving. Be sure you or your family member driving you home gets a chance to review the results of the colonoscopy with your doctor before you leave the endoscopy area. Knowing whether you have something to be concerned about or you're just expecting a letter to tell you to come back in ten years will be reassuring.

 Don't dedicate too much attention to worrying about biopsy results. Feel comfort knowing that you took the proper steps for your health by getting a colonoscopy and that you will take the proper steps for what happens next.

The fact is, colon cancer may be prevented if you undergo colonoscopy and have polyps removed before they turn into cancer. And if colon cancer does occur, it's curable when caught early. Doctors continue to discover more about colon cancer and the factors that influence its development, and as you're finding out, they also have effective screening tools that aid in its prevention.

Waiting for biopsy results

Waiting for your biopsy results to return from the laboratory can definitely cause stress. Relax, be patient, and read through these tips you can use to help handle that anxiety:

✔ Know what you can change and what you can't. Be flexible.

✔ Remember that the vast majority of polyps are noncancerous.

✔ Talk to people. Sharing your experience with friends or family may provide some laughs and may educate someone else.

✔ Laugh. Watch a funny movie, read a funny book, or hang out with funny friends. Laughter is good medicine.

✔ Have fun. Play a game with friends, a child, or a pet.

✔ Avoid stimulants. Coffee and cigarettes cause more stress than they relieve.

Chapter 7

Ten Common Questions

• •

In This Chapter

▶ Understanding why you need one

▶ Knowing what to expect

• •

*I*n this short chapter, I try to answer some common questions you may have about getting a colonoscopy. Knowing the answers to some of the questions can reduce your anxiety about having the procedure — I hope. Please read the questions, absorb the answers, and pass the message on to people who are still not convinced of the importance of a colonoscopy. Heck, tear out these pages and give it to them in a card . . . or just give them this book.

I tried to identify the questions most often asked, but I can't address every concern you may have. Your healthcare professionals can be a good resource when you have questions about this critical procedure. Do your best to get your questions answered and get screened today.

Why Do I Need to Get a Colonoscopy?

The simple answer is: Getting a colonoscopy can save your life. A colonoscopy can detect and remove polyps before they develop into colon cancer. It can also detect early stage colon cancer, if present, so it can be identified while still highly treatable. If you're 50 or older (or younger, with the risk factors discussed in Chapter 2) and have never had a screening colonoscopy, it's time. A common, simple procedure could save your life.

More than 90 percent of people diagnosed and treated when the cancer is confined to the colon or rectum survive more than five years. And according to the Centers for Disease Control and Prevention, 60 percent of deaths from colorectal cancer could be prevented if everyone age 50 and older were screened regularly.

When Should I Get My First Colonoscopy?

There are two types of colonoscopy:

- ✔ **Screening colonoscopy:** Schedule one of these when you reach the magic age of 50 (or 45 for African Americans) even if you don't have any symptoms. People with risk factors may need to start at a younger age.

- ✔ **Diagnostic colonoscopy:** Generally your doctor will recommend you have a colonoscopy if you exhibit certain symptoms or signs of potential colorectal polyps or cancer or other colon conditions. A diagnostic colonoscopy may be necessary at any age.

How Often Do I Need to Get a Colonoscopy for Colorectal Cancer Screening?

The good news is that, under normal circumstances, you only have to undergo a screening colonoscopy every ten years if the previous exam was normal and you don't have any other risk factors for colorectal cancer. And, who knows, by the time you need your next one, they may have figured out how to make the bowel prep taste good. (Chapter 4 talks about the prep process.) For individuals with an increased risk of colon polyps or cancer, the interval for colonoscopy can be shorter.

How Much Does It Cost and Will My Insurance Cover It?

The majority of insurance companies cover colorectal cancer screening, including colonoscopy. Thirty-two states have mandated insurance coverage for colonoscopy. However, your portion of the cost of colonoscopy varies greatly depending on your insurance coverage, where you have it done, and whether biopsies are performed or polyps are removed.

 Because the costs are so variable, if you're uninsured you should talk to your healthcare facility to discuss charges and payment options.

For more on the topic, see Chapter 1.

What Do I Have to Do to Get Ready?

It's not you, so much as your bowels, that need preparation for a colonoscopy. For the physician to get a good view of your colon lining, your bowel needs to be as empty and as clean as possible. To achieve this, your doctor will give you a prescription for a bowel prep, based on a discussion of your medical history and other medications you're taking, that will make you and your bathroom wallpaper good friends. (I talk about the prep process in Chapter 4.) Another very important issue prior to colonoscopy is following your doctor's instructions to adjust any medications that may make the procedure more hazardous or increase the risk for you if polyps need to be removed.

A helpful patient

A nurse tells a story about a patient who wanted to be more helpful than most. When she lifted the sheet to get him situated, there was a sign on the patient's bottom (in magic marker) "insert here" with an arrow pointing toward his anus!

Follow your doctor's instructions about recommendations for your medications, diet, and for getting your bowels cleaned out well in advance of the procedure. Contact your doctor if you have any questions or concerns about the instructions, the bowel prep you have been prescribed, or if you experience any unexpected problems during or after the prep. If you don't complete the preparation as instructed, your doctor may not be able to see your colon lining to detect abnormalities and you'll have wasted everyone's time and your money. The doctor will strongly recommend the procedure be repeated, maybe as soon as the next day. This means you must undergo yet another day of clear liquids, repeat the bowel prep, and ask a responsible adult for another ride home!

How Long Does the Procedure Take?

Most patients arrive about 30 minutes prior to the procedure to change clothes and get admitted to the pre-procedure room. Many people are surprised at how quickly the actual procedure flies by. Maybe it's the medicine. Maybe it's sleep deprivation. Maybe it's just that the procedure is really not that big a deal after all. It generally takes less than half an hour, and you most likely won't notice the time going by because you'll be under the influence of some calming drugs.

Does Getting a Colonoscopy Hurt?

Not generally. Most individuals are given conscious sedation or twilight sleep sedatives to make them very comfortable during the examination. Some people are amazed to be able to watch the exam and converse during it; however, many people wake up in the recovery room with little recollection of the procedures. Because the colon is collapsed into a series of folds, the doctor instills air to inflate it for a good view. The air may cause you to feel a little bloated or full during or after the procedure, but don't be ashamed to let it pass.

Your physician will provide you with a list of written discharge instructions including what symptoms may be normal after colonoscopy and what symptoms should prompt you to call them or seek urgent medical attention. If you experience severe abdominal pain, excessive rectal bleeding, fever, or anything unanticipated following the procedure, contact your healthcare provider as soon as possible. (For more on this topic, see Chapter 6.)

What Happens if the Doctor Finds Something Abnormal?

If your doctor finds polyps during the procedure, he or she can remove the majority of them right then and there using specialized tools called biopsy forceps or snares (looks like a lasso) that run inside the colonoscope.

If a polyp or tumor is too big to be safely removed through the colonoscope, the doctor will only sample the tissue to send to a lab to be tested under the microscope to determine the nature of the lesion. If other abnormalities are found in the colon, or the colonoscopy is being done to determine the cause of symptoms, biopsies can be performed.

Colonoscopy bingo!

A nurse had a conversation with an acquaintance several days after his procedure. The acquaintance thought his polyp was b-9 (like playing bingo), and was so proud to know the results. The nurse felt badly about correcting him, but was happy to deliver the good news: the polyp was benign. Ask the doctor to give you the results in writing!

It usually takes no more than one week to get the results of a biopsy. Your doctor will receive the report from the pathologist and then discuss the importance of the result with you. Important information to gather from your doctor includes the number, size, and pathology of polyps detected and the interval until the next colonoscopy should be scheduled.

How Long Does It Take to Recover?

Most people feel okay when they get into the recovery area. You may feel a bit groggy from the sedation/anesthesia and weak from the bowel prep process. For those and other reasons, you won't be allowed to leave the recovery room alone or drive yourself until the next day, so line up a ride ahead of time.

And with the bowel prep and the procedure itself, you'll probably not feel completely up to speed for the rest of the day. I recommend relaxing at home with some light food and lots of fluids and getting a good night's sleep so that you're ready to go the next morning. It's the perfect time to play the sympathy card with your significant other (or friends or family members)!

What Are the Alternatives to a Screening Colonoscopy?

The short answer is that a colonoscopy is by far the best, most thorough way to determine the cause of colon symptoms and to detect and remove colorectal polyps and cancer.

For colorectal cancer screening, other tests, including virtual colonoscopy, flexible sigmoidoscopy, fecal occult blood and DNA tests, and double contrast barium enema (DCBE) are other available screening tools. Each has its advantages and disadvantages. Generally however, if any abnormalities are uncovered with these alternative tests, you need a colonoscopy to confirm the findings and remove polyps, if present. (These procedures are discussed in Chapter 1.)

Chapter 8

Ten (Okay, Seven) Uncommon Questions

● ●

In This Chapter

▶ Discovering whether you can drink white wine

▶ Knowing whether to brush your teeth

● ●

*O*ver the years, many unique questions have been asked about colonoscopy, questions doctors don't hear every day. I can't even begin to list them all, but I wanted to share a few. Who knows, you might have been wondering about one of these! So here are some great not-so-frequently-asked-but-still-completely-valid questions.

Can I Drink White Wine While Prepping?

Well, technically white wine *is* a clear liquid, but a colonoscopy isn't a dinner party. Don't ever consume alcohol during the prep. Although your body will be churning out a lot of water, alcohol will increase the likelihood of dehydration. Dehydration is no fun. It's much more than just feeling "parched." It makes you feel really sick, and it's really dangerous. So keep the chardonnay chilled until well after your colonoscopy is complete and you're feeling back to normal. And, before you ask, this applies to beer, vodka, gin, or *any other* alcoholic beverage too.

Can I Wear Makeup or Jewelry During My Colonoscopy?

Makeup isn't going to make a bit of difference where the doctor will be looking. But if you're more comfortable when you're made up, there's no reason why you can't look nice for your big day . . . just don't let it make you late for your appointment! As far as jewelry, if you wear it to the facility, you may be told to remove it before the procedure.

Can I Have a Colonoscopy During My Period?

If this is a concern for you, talk to your doctor. But in the vast majority of cases, there won't be any issues with having a colonoscopy during a period. The prep may be more of a nuisance during your period, and some people may be embarrassed to provide such open access during this time, but being on your period isn't going to affect the ability to perform a successful colonoscopy or bowel preparation. And as far as the embarrassment issue, just know that healthcare professionals are used to dealing with the expected and unexpected. There's nothing to be worried about.

Can You Be Awake for a Colonoscopy?

Yes, you can be. It is a rare patient who prefers to undergo colonoscopy without any sedation, but even with sedation, not all patients go to sleep. Conscious sedation (covered in Chapter 5) usually leaves a patient in a dreamlike state and very comfortable for the procedure, but not truly "knocked out." Some people appear to be conscious, but they may not remember the exam afterwards. As mentioned before, it is possible to do the procedure without sedation, but unless there are extenuating factors, most patients appreciate and receive it.

Can You Have a Colonoscopy without a Prep?

No! There always needs to be some sort of colon preparation. It can be pretty messy in there, and without taking measures to clean the colon out, you're not putting yourself in the best position to catch anything abnormal that may be hiding.

Can Having a Colonoscopy Take off a Few Pounds?

Ah, wouldn't it be great if that were the case? An immediate lifestyle benefit from the torture you just endured. Unfortunately, it probably isn't going to happen. Despite what some of those shady colon cleanser ads claim, it is highly unlikely that you're carrying pounds and pounds of waste in your intestines. Colonoscopy isn't a diet strategy. Hate to break it to you, but nutrition and exercise are still the keys to weight loss.

Can I Brush My Teeth before a Colonoscopy?

If you are so inclined, please do. Your doctor and your staff will appreciate it!

Notes

Notes

Notes

Your Goal:
A CLEAN COLON
A clean colon is key to a successful colonoscopy

- A clean colon makes it easier for your doctor to identify abnormal growths that may be cancerous

- Follow your doctor's instructions to ensure your colon is as clean as possible (and avoid having your procedure canceled or repeated)

- Your doctor may recommend split dosing for your colonoscopy prep

What is split dosing?

This preparation strategy affects the timing of your prep medication. The first dosing series is taken the evening before your colonoscopy, and the second series is taken early on the morning of your colonoscopy. Waking up early to complete the prep is important because split dosing increases your chances for a cleaner colon before your colonoscopy.[1,2]

A cleaner colon provides a more accurate colonoscopy.

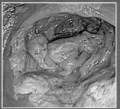

| Excellent prep | Good prep | Fair prep | Poor prep |

A fair or poor prep can leave the colon dirty, making it difficult for your doctor to spot abnormal growths. Following your doctor's directions may ensure a cleaner colon and a more accurate colonoscopy.

JUST SO YOU KNOW: The Importance of a Clean Colon
An informational resource brought to you by Salix Pharmaceuticals.

References: 1. Khan MA, Wasiuddin N, Brown M. Patient acceptance, convenience, and efficacy of one-day versus two-day colonoscopy bowel preparations. Poster presented at: Digestive Disease Week: May 20, 2008: San Diego, CA. **2.** Rex DK, Johnson DA, Anderson JC, Schoenfeld PS, Burke CA, Inadomi JM. American College of Gastroenterology guidelines for colorectal cancer screening 2008. *Am J Gastroenterol.* 2009;104:739-750.

HYDRATION
is essential for an effective colonoscopy prep

Taking a colonoscopy prep will cause you to lose fluids quickly—leading to dehydration

- Your fluids and minerals need to be replenished

- It is important to drink plenty of clear liquids before, during, and after the colonoscopy-prep process

- Follow your doctor's colonoscopy-prep directions very carefully

Drinking the recommended amount of liquid assists in the flushing process of prep medications and results in a more effective preparation. Most importantly, it keeps you hydrated. If you have any questions about how much to drink, ask your healthcare provider.

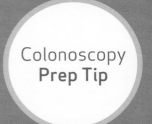

Colonoscopy Prep Tip

What is a clear liquid?

A clear liquid is any beverage you can see through that does not contain red or purple coloring. Examples of these could be: water, apple juice, ginger ale, lemon-lime soda, sports drink (eg, Gatorade®*), and lemonade.

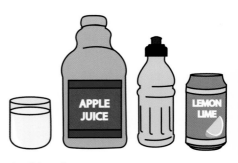

*Gatorade is a registered trademark of Stokely-Van Camp, Inc, Chicago, IL.

JUST SO YOU KNOW: The Importance of Hydration
An informational resource brought to you by Salix Pharmaceuticals.

 Salix Pharmaceuticals, Inc.   Web site: www.salix.com   1700 Perimeter Park Drive, Morrisville, NC 27560 Tel • 866.669.SLXP (7597)
©2011 Salix Pharmaceuticals, Inc.   All rights reserved. Printed in USA. SAL 11/04

You play the most important role in getting a clean colon

The few days before your colonoscopy are extremely important to ensure your colon is clean for optimal visibility during the procedure.

- ✓ **BEWARE OF OTHER MEDICINES.** Speak to your doctor about medicines that you may need to stop taking before your colonoscopy

- ✓ **WATCH WHAT YOU EAT.** Follow your doctor's recommendations about what you can and cannot eat before a colonoscopy

- ✓ **COMPLETE THE PREP.** Be sure to read all prep instructions, follow the recommendations for a precolonoscopy diet, and complete each step when instructed

- ✓ **STAY HYDRATED.** Be sure to drink all required liquids during the preparation, and replenish your system by drinking clear liquids after returning home from your colonoscopy

- ✓ **STAY NEAR A BATHROOM.** Many who have undergone colonoscopy preparation recommend the use of ointments and wet wipes to reduce the effects of many trips to the bathroom

- ✓ **SCHEDULE A RIDE HOME.** Because of the sedatives used during the colonoscopy, you will need someone to take you home

- ✓ **SPREAD THE WORD.** Make sure to tell those you know about the importance of getting screened—it could save a life

NOTE: No brochure can ever replace the advice of your healthcare team. Please carefully follow your doctor's instructions.

JUST SO YOU KNOW: Colonoscopy Prep Checklist
An informational resource brought to you by Salix Pharmaceuticals.

PASS ON
the importance of colon cancer screening

Colon cancer can affect you and your loved ones

- Colorectal cancer is the second leading cause of cancer-related death in the United States,[1] but it is preventable if the early warning signs are detected

- Because 90% of colorectal cancer cases occur in those aged 50 and older,[2] it's very important to take the preventative step of getting screened

A CALL FOR IMMEDIATE ACTION

If someone you care about is aged 50 or older, please pass on the importance of getting screened for colon cancer.

FREE INFORMATION
Encourage screening and alleviate fears in one easy read.

Download your free copy today!
www.ColonoscopyForDummies.com

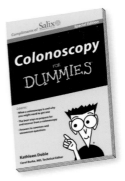

For Dummies is a registered trademark of Wiley Publishing, Inc.

References: 1. Foundation for Digestive Health and Nutrition. Colorectal cancer fact sheet. Available at: http://www.fdhn.org/wmspage.cfm?parm1=210. Accessed February 23, 2010. **2.** Colon Cancer Alliance. Disease information: CRC facts & figures. Available at: http://www.ccalliance.org/what_diseaseinfo_risk.html. Accessed February 23, 2010.

JUST SO YOU KNOW: Getting The Word Out
An informational resource brought to you by Salix Pharmaceuticals.

Salix Pharmaceuticals, Inc.
Web site: www.salix.com   1700 Perimeter Park Drive, Morrisville, NC 27560   Tel • 866.669.SLXP (7597)
©2011 Salix Pharmaceuticals, Inc.   All rights reserved.   Printed in USA.   SAL 11/03